BLOOD SUGAR

DIET

SOLUTION

The mastery method to overcome blood sugar imbalance and flourish by discovering the keys to changing health through a blood sugar diet

By

Johnny Gildon

Disclaimer

Copyright © 2022 Johnny Gildon. All Rights Reserved.

This book and its contents are protected by copyright law and may not be reproduced, distributed, transmitted, displayed, or otherwise published without the prior written permission from the copyright law.

Contents

Introduction

Chapter 1: Getting to Know Blood Sugar
-What is meant by blood sugar
-The Effects of Blood Sugar Levels on Health
-Typical Reasons for Elevated Blood Sugar

Chapter 2: The Low-Glycemic Diet
-What is a low glycemic diet
-The Advantages of Consuming Low-Glycemic Foods
-Foods to Include and Avoid on the Diet

Chapter 3: Recipes and Meal
-Planning Advice for the Blood Sugar Diet
-Sample Menus for Lunch, Dinner, and Breakfast
-Yummy and Healthful Low-Glycemic Dinner Recipes

Chapter 4: Physical Activity and Exercise
-Exercise Is Crucial Role in Blood Sugar Management
-Exercises Suggested for Blood Sugar Management
-Suggestions for Fitting Exercise Into Your Daily Schedule

Chapter 5: Monitoring Blood Sugar Levels

-How to Monitor Blood Sugar Levels at Home

-Comprehending Blood Glucose Levels

-When to Get Help for Abnormal Readings from a Doctor

Chapter 6: Strategies for Stress Reduction

-Stress's Effect on Blood Sugar Levels

-Techniques for Relaxation-Based Stress Management

-Stress-Reduction Breathing Techniques and Mindfulness Meditation

Chapter 7: Assistance and Responsibility

-Help Is Essential for Successfully Following the Blood Sugar Diet

-Collaborating with Registered Dietitians and Healthcare Providers

-Creating a Network of Support for Extended Success

Chapter 8: Modifying Your Lifestyle for Long-Term Success

-Advice on Changing Your Diet and Lifestyle in a Sustainable Way

-Creating reasonable objectives and monitoring advancement

-Honoring Achievements and Overcoming Obstacles

Summary of the Blood Sugar Diet Solution's Important Points

Blood sugar diet solution

Introduction

The Blood Sugar Diet Solution is a thorough program with scientific support that aims to assist people in efficiently controlling and optimizing their blood sugar levels for better health and overall well-being. This novel strategy lowers the risk of chronic illnesses including diabetes and cardiovascular disease by preventing insulin resistance, promoting stable blood sugar levels, and modifying lifestyle choices with the help of individualized assistance.

The Blood Sugar Diet Solution program offers a customized dietary plan that prioritizes whole foods high in fiber, lean proteins, healthy fats, and low-glycemic carbohydrates, all of which are adjusted to each participant's specific needs and goals. Through a focus on balanced meal planning and glycemic index education, participants are empowered to make choices that support stable blood sugar levels throughout the day.

Along with food recommendations, the Blood Sugar Diet Solution program stresses regular exercise as a way to support metabolic function, improve insulin sensitivity, and improve overall health. Individualized exercise regimens are encouraged to be incorporated into daily life to further optimize blood sugar control and cardiovascular fitness.

The Blood Sugar Diet Solution program's monitoring tools, continuing coaching or support from medical professionals, and frequent check-ins help participants stay on track and make sustainable progress toward optimal blood sugar management. People who adhere to the program's principles can reap several long-term health benefits, such as improved cardiovascular health, weight management, increased energy, decreased inflammation, improved cognitive function, and a lower risk of developing chronic diseases linked to unstable blood sugar levels.

In summary, the Blood Sugar Diet Solution program provides a comprehensive and useful approach to blood sugar control, enabling people to take charge of their health and well-being through customized assistance, lifestyle changes, and educated food choices. Participants can have a healthier and more active life, better control their blood sugar, and stop the course of disease by putting the principles taught in this program into practice.

Chapter 1: Getting to Know Blood Sugar

What is meant by blood sugar?

The concentration of glucose, a form of sugar, in the bloodstream, is referred to as blood sugar, often called blood glucose. The body uses glucose as one of its main energy sources for cells, and it is essential for many physiological functions. The body closely controls blood sugar levels to make sure cells have enough glucose available for synthesizing energy.

During digestion, carbohydrates (such as those found in bread, rice, fruits, and sweets) are converted into glucose and absorbed into the bloodstream. When blood sugar levels rise, the pancreas responds by releasing the hormone insulin. Insulin facilitates the movement of glucose into cells so that it can be stored for later use or used as fuel.

Keeping blood sugar levels steady is critical for general health and well-being. Blood sugar swings can have an instant impact on mood, energy levels, and cognitive abilities. Hyperglycemia, or persistently high blood sugar, can result in complications like diabetes, heart disease, nerve damage, and renal issues. Conversely, hypoglycemia, or low blood sugar, can result in symptoms including weakness, lightheadedness, disorientation, and even unconsciousness

People can maintain optimal health, prevent chronic diseases, and improve their overall quality of life by realizing the significance of blood sugar management and adopting lifestyle decisions that support stable blood sugar levels. Through dietary changes, increased physical activity, and other lifestyle interventions, the Blood Sugar Diet Solution program seeks to educate participants on practical methods for reducing blood sugar levels.

The Effects of Blood Sugar Levels on Health

Maintaining blood sugar levels is essential for general health and well-being. The body can operate at its best when blood sugar levels are well-regulated and within a healthy range. Blood sugar variations, however, can have a big effect on a lot of different parts of health.

The following are some ways that blood sugar levels can affect one's health:

Energy Levels: The body's cells, including those in the brain, primarily obtain their energy from glucose. Consistent blood sugar levels contribute to sustained high levels of energy throughout the day. Excessive or insufficient blood sugar levels can cause sensations of weakness, exhaustion, and poor energy.

Mood and Mental Health: Both mood and mental health are impacted by blood sugar levels. Fast variations in blood sugar, such as spikes or crashes, can cause impatience, anxiety, mood swings, and trouble focusing. Depression and cognitive decline may potentially be exacerbated by long-term blood sugar abnormalities.

Weight Management: The body's capacity to burn calories effectively and metabolism are both impacted by blood sugar levels. An ailment linked to weight gain and obesity, insulin resistance is brought on by high blood sugar levels. Low blood sugar, on the other hand, can cause cravings and hunger, which can result in overeating and weight gain.

Diabetes Risk: Hyperglycemia, or persistently elevated blood sugar, is a defining feature of diabetes. Diabetes that is not under control raises the chance of major side effects such as renal problems, nerve damage, cardiovascular disease, vision loss, and other health concerns. It is essential to keep blood sugar levels within normal ranges to prevent and treat diabetes.

Cardiovascular Health: High blood sugar raises the risk of heart disease and stroke by causing blood vessel damage. One significant risk factor for cardiovascular problems is persistent hyperglycemia. Making lifestyle changes to control blood sugar levels can help lower the risk of cardiovascular problems.

Inflammation and Immune Function: High blood sugar is associated with inflammation in the body, which is connected to several chronic illnesses, including autoimmune diseases, inflammatory bowel diseases, and arthritis. Additionally, long-term inflammation can impair immunity, leaving people more vulnerable to diseases and infections.

Neurological Health: Variations in blood sugar levels can affect cognitive and neurological health. Chronically elevated blood sugar levels have been linked to a higher risk of Alzheimer's disease, dementia, and cognitive decline. It is crucial to keep blood sugar levels steady to protect cognitive function and brain health.

People can improve their quality of life, lower their chance of developing chronic diseases, and promote general well-being by learning how blood sugar levels affect health and putting methods in place to maintain blood sugar levels stable. The Blood Sugar Diet Solution program offers advice on controlling blood sugar levels by using exercise, stress reduction, a healthy diet, and other lifestyle interventions.

Typical Reasons for Elevated Blood Sugar

Hyperglycemia, or elevated blood sugar, is brought on by several circumstances, such as:

Uncontrolled Diabetes: Uncontrolled diabetes is the most frequent cause of elevated blood sugar. The body does not generate insulin in type 1 diabetes, while it either produces insufficient insulin or develops resistance to its effects in type 2 diabetes. When there is insufficient insulin in the bloodstream to control blood sugar levels, glucose builds up and causes hyperglycemia.

Unhealthy Diet: Consuming unhealthy fats, refined carbs, and sugary foods and drinks in excess can cause blood sugar levels to rise. An unbalanced diet and insufficient fiber consumption can also lead to blood sugar fluctuations.

Insufficient Exercise: Engaging in regular physical exercise enhances insulin sensitivity and aids in the body's utilization of glucose for energy. Elevated blood sugar levels and insulin resistance can result from sedentary lifestyles.

Stress: Stress causes the body to generate substances that might elevate blood sugar, such as cortisol and adrenaline. Prolonged stress can interfere with the body's ability to produce and use insulin, which can result in elevated blood sugar levels.

Medication: As a side effect, various drugs, including diuretics, antipsychotics, corticosteroids, and some asthma treatments, might interfere with insulin function or raise blood sugar levels.

Illness or Infection: Conditions that result in inflammation or hormone abnormalities, as well as infections, can elevate blood sugar levels. Blood sugar spikes that are momentary may be caused by the body's reaction to an infection.

Hormonal Changes: High blood sugar levels and insulin sensitivity can be impacted by hormonal variations, which can happen during puberty, pregnancy, menopause, or disorders like polycystic ovarian syndrome (PCOS).

Sleep Deprivation: Poor sleep quality or insufficient sleep can interfere with hormone metabolism and regulation, which can result in insulin resistance and high blood sugar.

Alcohol Consumption: Drinking too much alcohol might damage the liver's ability to regulate glucose levels and cause brief rises in blood sugar levels.

Genetic Factors: The body's ability to process and control glucose may be influenced by genetic predisposition. People who have a family history of insulin resistance or diabetes may be more vulnerable to elevated blood sugar.

A combination of lifestyle changes, medication adherence (if needed), frequent monitoring, and consulting medical professionals are necessary to manage high blood sugar levels. People can better control their blood sugar levels and lower their risk of consequences from hyperglycemia by addressing the underlying causes of high blood sugar and forming healthy habits.

Chapter 2: The Low-Glycemic Diet

What is a low glycemic diet?

Consuming meals with little effect on blood sugar levels is the main goal of a low-glycemic diet, which helps control blood sugar levels and enhances general health. Foods are ranked on the glycemic index (GI) according to how rapidly they increase blood sugar levels after eating. Foods with a low GI value (55 or less) cause blood sugar levels to rise gradually because they take longer to digest and absorb.

A low-glycemic diet typically includes the following principles:

Focus on entire Foods: The foundation of a low-glycemic diet is entire, minimally processed foods such as fruits, vegetables, whole grains, legumes, nuts, and seeds. These meals help slow down digestion and stabilize blood sugar levels because they are high in fiber, vitamins, minerals, and antioxidants.

Healthful carbs: Select low-GI complex carbs from foods like sweet potatoes, yams, legumes (beans, lentils), and whole grains (oats, quinoa, brown rice). Because they digest more slowly than refined grains and sugars, these carbs help to minimize sudden rises in blood sugar levels.

Lean Proteins: Include low-fat dairy products, fish, chicken, tofu, and lentils in your meals as lean sources of protein. Protein increases satiety and aids in blood sugar regulation.

Good Fats: Include foods high in healthy fats in your diet, such as avocados, almonds, seeds, olive oil, and fatty fish (mackerel, salmon). Good fats can lower blood sugar levels by slowing down the absorption of carbohydrates.

Restrict Sugary Foods and Beverages: Restrict or stay away from high-GI foods and drinks such as soda, candies, baked goods, and cereals with added sugar. These products have the potential to quickly raise blood sugar levels.

Balanced Meals: To encourage consistent energy levels and avoid blood sugar swings, aim for balanced meals that contain a mix of carbs, proteins, and fats.

Portion Control: Be mindful of serving sizes to prevent overindulging, which may cause blood sugar levels to surge.

Regular Exercise: Exercise regularly to help control blood sugar levels and enhance insulin sensitivity.

A low-glycemic diet can help people control their blood sugar levels more effectively, lower their risk of insulin resistance and type 2 diabetes, and improve their general health and well-being. It is crucial to check with a healthcare physician or a trained dietitian before making large dietary changes to ensure that the diet is appropriate for individual health needs and objectives.

The Advantages of Consuming Low-Glycemic Foods

Consuming foods low in glucose has several health advantages, such as:

Stable Blood Sugar Levels: Foods with a low glycemic index take longer to digest and absorb, which causes blood sugar levels to rise gradually. This promotes more consistent blood sugar levels throughout the day by reducing blood sugar spikes and crashes.

Better Insulin Sensitivity: The body can more effectively control insulin levels when low-glycemic foods are consumed. This can lessen the chance of insulin resistance, increase insulin sensitivity, and decrease the chance of type 2 diabetes.

Weight Management: diets high in fiber and minerals, such as those found in low-glycemic diets, can help with feelings of fullness and satiety. This may support attempts to manage weight and lose weight by reducing overall calorie intake and controlling hunger.

Heart Health: Eating a lot of low-glycemic foods may be good for your heart. Low GI foods are frequently rich in fiber, antioxidants, and heart-healthy fats, all of which can lower cholesterol, lessen inflammation, and promote heart health.

Better Digestive Health: Low-glycemic, high-fiber foods can help with regular bowel movements, the maintenance of a healthy gut microbiome, and the prevention of diseases like diverticulosis and constipation.

Long-lasting Energy: Low-glycemic foods provide sustained energy levels due to their slow digestion and gradual release of glucose into the bloodstream. This can help prevent energy crashes and fatigue that may occur after consuming high-glycemic foods.

Reduced Risk of Chronic Diseases: Consuming a diet rich in low-glycemic foods has been associated with a lower risk of chronic diseases such as type 2 diabetes, cardiovascular disease, certain cancers, and metabolic syndrome.

Improved Mood and Mental Health: Stable blood sugar levels from low-glycemic foods can help regulate mood and energy levels. By avoiding blood sugar spikes and crashes, individuals may experience improved mental clarity, focus, and overall well-being.

Overall, incorporating more low-glycemic foods into your diet can have a positive impact on various aspects of health and may contribute to a balanced and sustainable approach to eating for long-term wellness. Foods to Include and Avoid on the Diet.

Foods to Include and Avoid on the Diet

When following a low-glycemic diet, it's important to focus on incorporating foods that have a low glycemic index (GI) and avoiding those with a high GI. Here are some meals to consider and steer clear of:

Foods to Consider

- **Non-Starchy Vegetables:** Broccoli, spinach, kale, cauliflower, bell peppers, zucchini, and other non-starchy vegetables are excellent choices as they are low in carbohydrates and have a low GI.

- **Legumes:** Beans, lentils, chickpeas, and other legumes are rich in fiber and protein, making them great options for a low-glycemic diet.

- **Whole Grains:** Choose whole grains like quinoa, barley, bulgur, and steel-cut oats over refined grains like white rice and white bread. These whole grains have a lower GI and provide more nutrients and fiber.

- **Nuts and Seeds:** Almonds, walnuts, chia seeds, flaxseeds, and other nuts and seeds are good sources of healthy fats, protein, and fiber with a low GI.

- **Healthy Fats:** Rich in monounsaturated fats and omega-3 fatty acids, avocado, olive oil, coconut oil, and fatty seafood like salmon can help regulate blood sugar levels.

- **Lean Proteins:** Skinless poultry, fish, tofu, tempeh, and eggs are good sources of protein with a low GI.

- **Low-Glycemic Fruits:** Berries (such as strawberries, blueberries, raspberries), apples, pears, and citrus fruits have a lower GI compared to tropical fruits like watermelon and pineapple.

- **Dairy:** Choose low-fat or non-fat dairy products like Greek yogurt, cottage cheese, and skim milk in moderation.

Foods to Steer Clear of

- **Highly Processed Foods:** Items with a high GI and high content of refined carbs include sugary snacks, sugary drinks, white bread, pastries, and fast food.
- **Sweetened Beverages:** Steer clear of sugar-filled beverages that can quickly raise blood sugar levels, such as soda, fruit juice, energy drinks, and sweetened teas.

- **White Potatoes:** Because of their high carbohydrate content, white potatoes have a high GI. Sweet potatoes or other root vegetables are a better option.

- **White Rice and Pasta:** Refined grains with their fiber extracted during processing, such as white rice and pasta, have a higher GI. Opt instead for whole-grain substitutes.

- **Candy and Sweets:** Steer clear of sugary items that might spike blood sugar levels, such as cakes, cookies, and candy.

- **Processed Meats:** Meats that have been processed, such as hot dogs, sausages, and deli meats, may have fillers or additional sugars that might affect blood sugar levels.

You may design a well-rounded low-glycemic diet that promotes general health and well-being by concentrating on whole, minimally processed foods with a low GI and balancing your meals with a balance of lean proteins, healthy fats, fiber-rich carbohydrates, and an abundance of veggies.

Chapter 3: Recipes and Meal

Planning Advice for the Blood Sugar Diet

The blood sugar diet relies heavily on meal planning since it keeps you on track with your nutritional objectives and guarantees that you eat a balanced diet every day of the week. On the blood sugar diet, the following advice can help with meal planning:

Plan Ahead: Allocate a portion of your weekly schedule to organize your meals for the following days. This might assist you in choosing better options and preventing impulsive judgments that might conflict with your nutritional objectives.

Incorporate a Variety of Foods: Try to incorporate a range of foods, such as whole grains, lean proteins, healthy fats, and an abundance of veggies, into your meal plan. By doing this, you can make sure that the nutrients and flavors in your food are being balanced well.

Put an Emphasis on Low-Glycemic Foods: To help regulate blood sugar levels, choose foods with a low glycemic index (GI). Make sure your meals contain an abundance of lean meats, legumes, whole grains, nuts, and seeds in addition to non-starchy vegetables.

Prepare Ingredients Ahead of Time: If you want to save time during the week, think about preparing ingredients ahead of time. To make meal preparation easier when it is time to eat, chop vegetables, cook grains, and prepare proteins in advance.

Batch Cook: Take into account preparing some meals, or parts of meals, in bulk, like stews, soups, and roasted vegetables. This can benefit you when you're pressed for time by having nutritious selections close at hand.

Portion Control: When organizing your meals, consider the proportions of the portions. Measure out portions and prevent overeating by using food scales, measuring cups, or visual cues (such as using your hand as a guide).

Incorporate Snacks: To help stave off hunger and avoid overindulging during main meals, schedule nutritious snacks in between meals. Choose high-protein, high-fiber, and healthy-fat snacks to help control blood sugar levels.

Remain Hydrated: Remember to factor in hydration when you plan your meals. Make sure to stay hydrated throughout the day, and for some extra taste, try adding herbal teas or infused water.

Listen to Your Body: Observe how different foods impact your energy and blood sugar levels. As your body reacts to different foods, make necessary adjustments to your diet plan.

Seek Support: To assist you in developing a customized meal plan that complements your unique health objectives and is in line with the blood sugar diet, think about consulting with a licensed dietitian or nutritionist.

You can prepare healthy, well-balanced meals that promote stable blood sugar levels and general well-being while following a blood sugar diet by using these suggestions in your meal planning process.

Sample Menus for Lunch, Dinner, and Breakfast

The following are some examples of blood sugar diet-compliant breakfast, lunch, and dinner menus:

Breakfast:
- Eggs scrambled with cherry tomatoes and spinach
- Avocado on whole-grain bread
- Dark coffee or herbal tea

Lunch:
- A salad of grilled chicken topped with bell peppers, cucumbers, mixed greens, and vinaigrette dressing
- Feta cheese, cherry tomatoes, and chickpeas in quinoa salad

- Water with lemon or iced tea without sugar

Dinner:
- Tofu stir-fried with broccoli, bell peppers, and snap peas in a light soy sauce
- Baked fish with roasted asparagus and quinoa
- A dessert of mixed berry salad drizzled with balsamic vinegar

On the blood sugar diet, these sample meal plans include a decent combination of whole grains, lean meats, healthy fats, and an abundance of veggies to support stable blood sugar levels and general health. You are welcome to modify the amounts and components to suit your nutritional requirements and tastes.

Yummy and Healthful Low-Glycemic Dinner Recipes

Here are three low-glycemic meals that are both tasty and nourishing that you may try:

Roasted Vegetables and Baked Lemon Herb Chicken:

Ingredients
- 4 skinless, boneless chicken breasts
- 1 lemon, squeezed and zesting
- 2 chopped garlic cloves
- 1 teaspoon of oregano, dried
- A teaspoon of thyme, dried

- 2 cups of mixed vegetables (such as bell peppers, zucchini, and cherry tomatoes)
- Salt and pepper to taste
- 2 tablespoons olive oil

Guidelines

1. Set the oven's temperature to 400°F or 200°C.

2. Combine the lemon juice, zest, garlic, oregano, thyme, salt, and pepper in a small bowl.

3. Transfer the chicken breasts to a baking sheet and cover them with the herb-lemon mixture. Allow to steep for thirty minutes.

4. In the baking dish, arrange the mixed veggies around the chicken. Add salt,

pepper, and a dash of olive oil for seasoning.

5. Bake for 25 to 30 minutes, or until the chicken is thoroughly cooked and the vegetables are soft, in a preheated oven.

Ingredients for Lentil and Vegetable Soup:

- 1 cup of rinsed brown or green lentils
- 1 chopped onion
- 2 diced carrots
- 2 diced celery stalks
- 2 minced garlic cloves
- 1 teaspoon of paprika and cumin each
- 4 cups vegetable broth
- To taste, salt and pepper
- Garnish with fresh parsley

Instructions

1. Sauté the onion, carrots, celery, and garlic in olive oil in a large pot until they soften.

2. Add the lentils, cumin, paprika, and vegetable broth to the pot. Bring to a boil, then lower the heat and simmer the lentils until they are tender about 20 to 25 minutes.

3. To taste, add more salt and pepper.

4. Serve hot, garnished with fresh parsley.

Ingredients for Grilled Salmon with Quinoa Salad and Asparagus:

- 4 salmon filets

- 1 bunch of trimmed asparagus
- 1 cup cooked quinoa, following package directions
- 1 diced red bell pepper
- 1/4 cup chopped fresh parsley
- 1 lemon juice
- 2 tablespoons olive oil
- salt and pepper to taste.

Instructions

1. Increase the temperature of a grill or grill pan to medium-high.

2. Use salt and pepper to season the salmon fillets. Cook on the grill for 4–5 minutes on each side, or until well done.

3. Combine salt, pepper, and olive oil with the asparagus. Grill until soft, about 3–4 minutes.

4. Put the cooked quinoa, chopped parsley, diced red bell pepper, olive oil, lemon juice, salt, and pepper in a big bowl. 5. Present the asparagus and grilled salmon over quinoa salad.

These meals are great for anyone on a blood sugar diet or trying to control their blood sugar levels because they're low-glycemic and delicious.

Chapter 4: Physical Activity and Exercise

Exercise Is Crucial Role in Blood Sugar Management

Exercise is essential for controlling blood sugar levels in those with diabetes or those who are at risk of getting the disease. The following are some main justifications for the significance of exercise in blood sugar regulation:

Enhances Insulin Sensitivity: Exercise regularly makes the body more receptive to insulin, the hormone that controls blood sugar levels. This implies that insulin will be used by the body more efficiently to move glucose from the bloodstream into the cells where it is needed for energy.

Lowers Blood Sugar Levels: By boosting the muscles' absorption of glucose for energy both during and after physical activity, exercise helps lower blood sugar levels. This may result in lower blood sugar levels generally, particularly for those who have type 2 diabetes.

Aids in Weight Management: Maintaining a healthy weight is important for managing blood sugar levels, as excess body weight can lead to insulin resistance and elevated blood sugar levels.

Lowers Risk of Complications: Regular physical activity can help lower the risk of complications associated with diabetes, such as heart disease, stroke, nerve damage, and kidney disease. By controlling blood sugar levels through exercise, people can lower their risk of developing these complications.

Increases Cardiovascular Health: Exercise is beneficial for general cardiovascular health, including increasing heart function, reducing blood pressure, and lowering cholesterol levels. These characteristics are significant for those with diabetes, as they are at a higher risk of cardiovascular disease.

Improves Mood and Mental Health: Research has indicated that physical activity is beneficial for mental health and overall well-being. It can aid in lowering depression, anxiety, and stress—all of which are typical issues for people with diabetes. A cheerful outlook might also help with maintaining a healthy lifestyle more consistently.

Improves General Fitness: Engaging in regular physical exercise can raise one's degree of general fitness, which includes balance, strength, flexibility, and endurance. Better quality of life and an increased capacity to carry out daily tasks with ease can result from this.

In summary, exercise is an effective strategy for controlling blood sugar levels and enhancing general health in people with diabetes or at risk for the disease. To get the most results, it is advised to combine strength training activities with aerobic activity (such as walking, cycling, or swimming). See a doctor before starting a new exercise regimen, particularly if you have any underlying medical conditions.

Exercises Suggested for Blood Sugar Management

For people with diabetes or those at risk of developing the disease, various forms of exercise are advised for controlling blood sugar levels and enhancing general health. The following are some essential forms of exercise that are good for controlling blood sugar:

Aerobic Exercise: Also referred to as cardio exercise, aerobic exercise entails actions that quicken breathing and heart rate. Because this kind of activity facilitates the body's utilization of glucose for energy, it is very helpful in reducing blood sugar levels. Walking, jogging, cycling, swimming, dancing, and aerobics classes are a few aerobic exercise options.

Strength Training: Strength training exercises, also known as resistance or weight-bearing exercises, involve using weights, resistance bands, or your body weight to build muscle strength. Strength training can help improve insulin sensitivity and glucose uptake by muscles, leading to better blood sugar control. Examples of strength training exercises include weightlifting, bodyweight exercises (e.g., push-ups, squats), and using resistance bands.

Flexibility and Balance Exercises: Flexibility and balance exercises are important for overall fitness and can help prevent injuries. Activities such as yoga, Pilates, tai chi, and stretching exercises can improve flexibility, balance, and coordination. These exercises can also help reduce stress and promote relaxation, which can have a positive impact on blood sugar levels.

Interval Training: In interval training, high-intensity workouts are interspersed with low-intensity recuperation sessions. This kind of activity has the potential to increase insulin sensitivity, burn calories, and improve cardiovascular fitness. You can perform interval training using a variety of exercises, including bodyweight movements, cycling, and running.

Mind-Body Exercises: These exercises emphasize the relationship between the mind and body and can help with stress management, relaxation, and general well-being. Blood sugar regulation may be positively impacted by stress management practices such as deep breathing exercises, mindfulness, meditation, and relaxation techniques.

Low-Impact Activities: Low-impact exercises like stationary bike, water aerobics, and walking on flat surfaces might be helpful for people with joint discomfort or mobility problems. These exercises improve general health and circulation while offering a more mild workout.

Daily Exercise: Including regular exercise in your routine is crucial for controlling blood sugar levels. Easy things like walking during work breaks, gardening, playing with pets, and using the stairs instead of the elevator can help improve blood sugar control and general physical fitness.

Before beginning a new workout program, it's crucial to speak with a healthcare physician or a trained fitness professional, particularly if you have any underlying medical ailments or concerns. They can provide customized guidance based on your unique needs and goals. To prevent damage and to get the most out of exercise for blood sugar control, always start carefully, pay attention to your body, and then progressively increase the intensity and duration of your workouts.

Suggestions for Fitting Exercise Into Your Daily Schedule

It's not necessary to make exercise a complicated or time-consuming part of your daily routine. Here are some tips to help you make exercise a regular part of your day:

Set Realistic Goals: Whether your goal is to commit to a specific workout routine, walk a certain number of steps a day, or take more breaks during the day, having clear goals can help you stay motivated.

Find Activities You Enjoy: Whether your activity is dancing, hiking, biking, swimming, or playing a sport, finding activities that you enjoy and look forward to doing will make it easier to stick with them over time.

Establish a Habit: Plan your physical activities and workouts the same way you would any other appointment or commitment. When it comes to creating a habit, consistency is essential, so make an effort to create a routine that you enjoy.

Break It Up: If scheduling a lengthy workout seems difficult, divide your exercise into shorter bursts throughout the day. Exercise, even for just ten to fifteen minutes each day, can build up and have health advantages.

Be Active Throughout the Day: Seek opportunities to move throughout the day, such as parking further away from your destination, using the stairs instead of the elevator, or performing domestic duties that call for movement.

Mix It Up: Change things up by trying new things. Try strength training, cardio, and flexibility exercises. Enroll in fitness classes. Go outside and do activities.

Involve Others: Work out with a friend, family member, or group to stay accountable and motivated. Working out with a workout partner can make it more fun and provide social support.

Use Technology: Use fitness apps, activity trackers, or smart devices to monitor your progress, set goals, and track your workouts. These tools can help you stay on track and provide motivation to reach your fitness objectives.

Reward Yourself: Commemorate your victories and life achievements. Reward yourself for keeping active and making progress. It could be as simple as getting a massage, purchasing new exercise equipment, or treating yourself to a nutritious snack.

Listen to Your Body: Observe the sensations that exercise causes in your body, both during and after. If you feel pain or discomfort, stop and speak with a medical practitioner or fitness expert. It's crucial to exercise sensibly and refrain from overexerting yourself.

Remember that every little bit of movement counts, so don't be too hard on yourself if you miss a workout or have a busy day. The key is to stay consistent, listen to your body, and make physical activity a priority for your overall health and well-being.

Chapter 5: Monitoring Blood Sugar Levels

How to Monitor Blood Sugar Levels at Home

A vital component of managing diabetes and maintaining good health is home blood sugar monitoring. The following steps will assist you in effectively monitoring your blood sugar levels:

Select a Blood Glucose Monitor: There are a variety of blood glucose monitors on the market. Discuss with your healthcare provider which one is best for you based on your needs, lifestyle, and insurance coverage.

Read the Instructions: Make sure you understand how to use your blood glucose monitor by carefully reading the instructions that come with it. If you have any questions, don't be afraid to ask your healthcare provider or a pharmacist.

Wash Your Hands: Use soap and water to wash your hands before doing a blood sugar test in order to get rid of any debris, food residue, or other materials that can skew the results.

Establish the Testing Area: Ensure that all the items you'll need are at hand, such as alcohol swabs, test strips, lancets, and a sharps container for the safe disposal of lancets.

Prepare the Lancet Device: Insert a lancet into the lancet device according to the manufacturer's instructions. If required, change the lancet device's depth setting.

Insert a Test Strip: Follow the instructions to insert a test strip into the meter. Ensure the meter is ready to take the test strip and that it is turned on.

Prick Your Finger: Prick the side of your fingertip using the lancet gadget. Gently press your finger to generate a tiny droplet of blood.

Apply Blood to Test Strip: Touch the test strip's edge to your fingertip's blood drop. After analyzing the blood sample, the meter will show your blood sugar level on the screen.

Document Your Findings: Maintain a record of your blood sugar measurements, together with the time, date, and associated values. Together, you and your healthcare provider can use this information to identify trends and, if necessary, modify your treatment strategy.

Act on the Results: If your blood sugar is too high or too low, follow your doctor's recommendations for changing your diet, medication, or amount of physical activity.

Clean Up: To prevent infection, dispose of the lancet and test strip safely in a sharps container and wash your hands again.

Regularly Review Your Data: Review your blood sugar logs with your doctor on a regular basis to monitor your progress, spot trends, and make any necessary adjustments to your diabetes management plan.

You may actively manage your diabetes and keep yourself healthy by adhering to these guidelines and routinely checking your blood sugar levels. Consult your healthcare practitioner for advice and assistance if you have any questions or concerns about checking your blood sugar levels at home.

Comprehending Blood Glucose Levels

In order to effectively manage your diabetes, it is important that you understand your blood glucose readings. The following points will help you interpret your blood glucose levels:

Normal Blood Glucose Levels: After eating, blood sugar levels may rise, but they should usually return to normal within a few hours.

Target Blood Glucose Range: Your healthcare provider will determine a target range for your blood sugar levels based on factors like your age, overall health, and type of diabetes. Typically, a target range for fasting blood sugar is between 80 and 130 mg/dL, and a target range for postprandial (after-meal) blood sugar is below 180 mg/dL.

Hyperglycemia, or High Blood Glucose: If your blood sugar levels are routinely higher than the recommended range, you may have hyperglycemia. Increased thirst, frequent urination, exhaustion, impaired vision, and sluggish wound healing are signs of elevated blood sugar. If high blood sugar is not appropriately controlled, problems may arise.

Low Blood Sugar (Hypoglycemia): Hypoglycemia is a condition in which your blood sugar falls below normal range (below 70 mg/dL). Low blood sugar manifests as trembling, perspiration, disorientation, lightheadedness, and hunger. Hypoglycemia severe enough to cause convulsions or unconsciousness.

Interpreting Patterns: You can spot trends and patterns by routinely checking your blood sugar levels. For instance, you could observe that, after particular meals or during particular times of the day, your blood sugar levels are constantly elevated. You can use this information to help you make changes to your medication, food, or lifestyle.

Speak with Your Healthcare Provider: It's critical to speak with your healthcare provider if you have any questions regarding your blood sugar readings or if you observe recurring trends of high or low blood sugar levels. They can assist you in comprehending the findings, modifying your medication plan as needed, and provide advice on how to properly manage your diabetes.

Make Use of Resources: To assist you in better understanding and managing your blood glucose levels, your healthcare practitioner may suggest extra resources, such as diabetes educators or nutritionists. These experts can offer helpful advice and assistance to improve your treatment of diabetes.

You can take proactive measures to maintain optimal blood sugar control, lower the risk of complications, and live a better life with diabetes by learning how to correctly interpret and comprehend your blood glucose levels. Successful management of diabetes requires regular monitoring, contact with your healthcare team, and lifestyle changes.

When to Get Help for Abnormal Readings from a Doctor

It is imperative that you get medical assistance if you have abnormal blood glucose readings in order to effectively manage your diabetes and avoid complications. When to seek medical attention for aberrant readings, according to the following guidelines:

Persistently High Blood Sugar Levels: It's critical to get in touch with your healthcare practitioner if, even after adhering to your treatment plan, your blood sugar levels continue to be higher than your goal range. Hyperglycemia, or persistently high blood sugar, can cause long-term consequences such as kidney damage, nerve damage, and cardiovascular problems.

Severe Hyperglycemia Symptoms: Get medical help right away if you suffer from severe hyperglycemia symptoms, which include intense thirst, frequent urination, disorientation, or trouble breathing. These signs could point to a medical emergency that needs to be attended to right now.

Low Blood Glucose Levels: If your blood sugar levels drop below 70 mg/dL and you feel symptoms of hypoglycemia, such as shakiness, sweating, confusion, or loss of consciousness, take immediate steps to increase your blood sugar level. If symptoms persist or worsen, seek medical attention soon.

Recurrent Hypoglycemia: See your doctor if, despite treatment plan modifications, you often have low blood sugar episodes. Recurrent hypoglycemia can be harmful and might mean that your drug regimen or way of living needs to be adjusted.

Unexplained Fluctuations: It's critical to talk to your healthcare professional about any abrupt or unexplained variations in your blood sugar levels. They can suggest suitable changes and assist in determining possible causes, such as food issues, stress, illness, or drug combinations.

New Symptoms or Concerns: Please contact your healthcare team without delay if you experience any new diabetes-related symptoms or if you have questions about your blood glucose readings. Early problem-solving and avoidance can be achieved by prompt communication.

Changes in General Health: Notify your healthcare practitioner of any notable changes in your general health, such as an inexplicable weight loss, recurring infections, or unusual exhaustion. Your treatment plan may need to be modified as a result of these changes, which may affect how you manage your diabetes.

Recall that maintaining optimal blood glucose control and managing your diabetes effectively require timely communication with your healthcare professional. You may improve your health and quality of life with diabetes by getting help when you need it and taking an active role in your care.

Chapter 6: Strategies for Stress Reduction

Stress's Effect on Blood Sugar Levels

Blood sugar levels can be significantly impacted by stress, particularly in those who have diabetes. Blood sugar levels may rise as a result of the hormones your body releases during stress, such as cortisol and adrenaline. This is your body's "fight or flight" response, meant to react to a perceived threat. The following are some ways that stress may impact a diabetic's blood sugar levels:

Increased Insulin Resistance: Stress hormones can increase your cells' resistance to the effects of insulin, the hormone that controls blood sugar levels. Higher blood sugar levels may result from your body's inability to properly use glucose.

Modifications in Eating Patterns: Stress can also affect how you eat, causing you to eat emotionally, crave high-fat or high-sugar foods, or skip meals. These dietary modifications may affect the regulation of blood sugar and cause variations in glucose levels.

Levels of Physical Activity: Stress might make it harder for you to feel motivated to work out or be physically active, which can interfere with your body's capacity to control blood sugar. Maintaining stable blood sugar levels and treating diabetes need regular exercise.

Medication Adherence: Stress has been shown to have an impact on people's ability to follow prescription regimens, check-in times, and general self-care procedures. Uncontrolled glucose levels might result from missing medication doses or from not checking your blood sugar regularly.

Sleep Disturbances: Stress can throw off your sleep cycles, leaving you with insufficient rest and possibly hormone imbalances. Inadequate sleep can affect blood sugar regulation and worsen complications associated with diabetes. **Prolonged or Chronic Stress:** Managing stress with mindfulness exercises, relaxation techniques, or seeking help from medical professionals or mental health specialists is essential for maintaining optimal glucose control. Over time, prolonged or chronic stress can have a more significant effect on blood sugar levels.

Take into account the following tactics to control how stress affects blood sugar levels:

- Engage in stress-relieving exercises like yoga, meditation, deep breathing, or mindfulness.

- Keep up a healthy lifestyle by getting enough sleep, eating a balanced diet, and engaging in regular physical activity.

- Communicate openly with your healthcare team about pressures and concerns connected to diabetes control.

- To deal with stress and emotional difficulties, ask friends, family, or support groups for assistance.

- Take into account therapy or counseling to address underlying stressors and create coping skills.

You can help yourself feel better overall and manage your diabetes more effectively if you take proactive measures to reduce stress and its effects on blood sugar levels. Recall that lowering the risk of complications from diabetes and preserving stable blood sugar control depend heavily on stress management.

Techniques for Relaxation-Based Stress Management

Reducing stress and elevating general wellbeing can both be accomplished with the use of relaxation techniques. Here are some tactics that you may implement:

Deep Breathing: To relax your body and mind, engage in deep breathing exercises. Breathe in deeply and slowly via your nose for a few seconds, then release the air gently through your mouth. To encourage relaxation and lessen stress, repeat this multiple times.

Progressive Muscle Relaxation: This method has you tensing and relaxing various bodily muscle groups. Beginning at your toes and working your way up to your head, give each muscle group a brief period of attention before letting go of any tightness. This can reduce bodily tension and encourage calmness.

Mindfulness Meditation: Practice mindfulness meditation to develop a calmer mind and a greater awareness of the present moment. To help you stay in the now and de-stress, pay attention to your breathing, your body's feelings, or the sounds around you.

Yoga: By incorporating physical postures, breathing techniques, and meditation, yoga can help reduce stress. Yoga encourages awareness, relaxation, and flexibility, all of which are beneficial to your physical and mental health.

Guided Imagery: To conjure up an image in your mind of a tranquil and soothing setting, use guided imagery or visualization techniques. To relax and relieve tension, close your eyes, picture yourself in a peaceful setting, and concentrate on the sights, sounds, and feelings there.

Aromatherapy: To induce calmness and relaxation, use essential oils such as bergamot, lavender, or chamomile. To feel the calming effects of essential oils, diffuse them, add them to a bath, or use them physically.

Journaling: To process emotions and lower stress, write down your thoughts, feelings, and experiences in a journal. Writing about oneself can assist you in gaining perspective, recognizing stressors, and creating coping mechanisms.

Physical Activity: To release endorphins and lower stress levels, regularly engage in physical activity like walking, running, dancing, or cycling. Physical activity is an organic way to reduce stress and enhance mood as well as general wellbeing.

Listening to Music: To decompress, play some soothing music or take in some natural sounds. Music is a simple yet powerful stress-reduction tool because of its ability to affect emotions and encourage relaxation.

Reconnecting with Nature: To relax, decompress, and rejuvenate, spend time in the great outdoors. To encourage calm and relaxation, go for a stroll in a park, have a seat by the water, or just take in the beauty of the natural world.

You can improve your overall quality of life, efficiently manage stress, and lower blood sugar levels by implementing these relaxing techniques into your regular routine. Try out various tactics to see which ones work best for you, and prioritize taking care of yourself in order to manage stress associated with diabetes.

Stress-Reduction Breathing Techniques and Mindfulness Meditation

Breathing techniques and mindfulness meditation are effective methods for reducing stress and promoting general well-being. Here's how to apply these routines to your everyday life:

Meditation with mindfulness:

1. Look for a peaceful, distraction-free area where you can sit or lie down.
2. Shut your eyes and concentrate on your breathing. Observe the sensation of each inhaled and exhaled breath.
3. Gently return your attention, without passing judgment, to your breathing if your thoughts stray.
4. Increase the range of sensations you are aware of, including your body's feelings, the sounds around you, and your thoughts.
5. Spend a few minutes each day practicing mindfulness meditation. As you get more accustomed to the technique, you can progressively extend the time.

Breathing Techniques:

Deep breathing: Take a seat or lie down in a comfortable posture. Put your hands on your abdomen and your chest, respectively. Breathe in deeply through your nose, filling up your belly, and then gently release the air through your mouth. To de-stress and soothe your nervous system, repeat this multiple times.

4-7-8 Breathing: Take a 4-count breath via your nose, hold it for a 7-count breath, then release it through your mouth for an 8-count. This breathing technique can ease anxiety, encourage relaxation, and help you control your breathing.

Box Breathing: Take a deep breath, hold it for 4 counts, exhale for 4 counts, and then hold it for 4 more counts before beginning the cycle again. Continue breathing in this manner to help your body and mind relax.

Regularly engaging in breathing exercises and mindfulness meditation can help you develop a sense of calm, lower stress levels, and enhance your general well-being. These methods can be effective tools for improving your quality of life, reducing stress, and encouraging relaxation. Try out many techniques to see which ones are most effective for you, and prioritize self-care in your everyday activities.

Chapter 7: Assistance and Responsibility

Help Is Essential for Successfully Following the Blood Sugar Diet

Success on the Blood Sugar Diet, or any health-related journey, is mostly dependent on support. Here are some explanations for why assistance is crucial:

Accountability and Motivation: Having a solid support network can help you stay accountable and motivated. It might be encouraging to know that people are holding you accountable and supporting you while you make dietary and lifestyle adjustments.

Emotional Support: Changing your food and way of life can be difficult. You can deal with any emotional ups and downs that may occur during your journey by getting emotional support from friends, family, or a support group.

Practical Support: Help can also take the shape of helping out with tasks like grocery shopping, meal planning, or preparing nutritious meals together. It may be simpler for you to maintain your diet and make better decisions with this helpful assistance.

Sharing Experiences: Making connections with people who are on the Blood Sugar Diet can give you a sense of belonging and enable you to exchange success stories, advice, and tactics. Getting knowledge from those who have gone through comparable events can be beneficial for your path.

Celebrating Successes: Rewarding yourself and your community for any accomplishment, no matter how tiny, will give you more self-assurance and drive to keep improving your health.

Expert counsel: Seeking assistance from medical professionals, dietitians, or other experts can offer you individualized counsel and support to help you succeed on the Blood Sugar Diet, in addition to peer support.

All things considered, following the Blood Sugar Diet and reaching your health objectives can be greatly impacted by having a solid support network. Finding support that suits you, whether from friends, family, internet forums, or medical professionals, can improve your path to improved health and well-being.

Collaborating with Registered Dietitians and Healthcare Providers

When adhering to the Blood Sugar Diet or any other health-related program, it might be quite helpful to collaborate with medical professionals and certified dietitians. The following are some justifications for why consulting these experts is crucial:

Individualized advice: Based on your unique health needs, medical history, and goals, registered dietitians and healthcare professionals can offer individualized advice. They may assist in customizing the Blood Sugar Diet to meet your unique needs and guarantee that you are adhering to a secure and efficient diet.

Medical Monitoring: It's critical to collaborate with healthcare specialists to evaluate your progress and make necessary adjustments if you take medication or have underlying health concerns. They can assist in making sure that you are improving healthily and that the diet is in line with your requirements.

Nutritional Expertise: Trained specialists in nutrition, and registered dietitians may offer professional guidance on how to improve your diet for blood sugar regulation, weight control, and general health. They may assist you in developing balanced meal plans, making better decisions, and comprehending the nutritional value of various foods.

Behavioral Support: To assist you in overcoming obstacles, forming healthy habits, and maintaining motivation along your journey, registered dietitians and healthcare professionals can also give behavioral support. They can offer methods for controlling cravings, handling stress, and implementing long-term lifestyle adjustments.

Tracking Progress: Visiting doctors and nutritionists regularly will help you monitor your progress, spot possible problems, and make any required plan modifications. Key health indicators, like weight, cholesterol, and blood sugar levels, can be measured to make sure you are on the correct route.

Safety: You can make sure you are following the Blood Sugar Diet safely and successfully by collaborating with medical professionals and certified dietitians. They can offer advice on possible dangers, adverse effects, and contraindications. They can also step in if there are any issues.

In general, you can improve your experience and chances of success on the Blood Sugar Diet by working with medical professionals and trained dietitians. Their knowledge, direction, and assistance can help you overcome the obstacles of altering your food and way of life while achieving the best possible results for your health.

Creating a Network of Support for Extended Success

Creating a solid support network is essential for long-term success while implementing any health-related program, including the Blood Sugar Diet. Here are some pointers for setting up a nurturing environment that will aid in keeping you inspired and on course:

Involve Family and Friends: Tell your loved ones about your objectives and difficulties. Tell them how they can help you, whether it's by preparing nutritious meals with you, participating in physical activities with you, or just lending a supportive word.

Join a Support Group: If you're following the Blood Sugar Diet, you might want to consider joining an online community or support group. Making connections with people who are traveling the same path as you can offer support, accountability, and inspiration.

Consult a Health Coach: If you would rather get one-on-one assistance, you might want to look into hiring a health coach, who can offer individualized direction, inspiration, and accountability. A health coach can assist you in establishing reasonable objectives, monitoring your development, and overcoming setbacks.

Seek Professional Advice: As previously indicated, consulting with registered dietitians and healthcare professionals can provide insightful knowledge and assistance. They may offer you tailored guidance, keep an eye on your development, and support you through any obstacles that could come up.

Set Achievable and practical Goals: Make sure your short- and long-term goals are both attainable and practical. To keep yourself encouraged and motivated to keep working for your ultimate health objectives, acknowledge and celebrate your tiny accomplishments along the way.

Establish a Positive Environment: As you embark on your road toward health and well-being, surround yourself with supportive people. This may be clearing out bad foods from your cupboard, coming up with new stress-reduction techniques, or introducing mindfulness exercises into your everyday routine.

Track Your Progress: Keep tabs on important health indicators, like blood sugar, weight, and energy levels, to stay informed about your progress. By keeping track of your progress, you can hold yourself more accountable and make the necessary corrections to continue on course.

Exercise Self-Care: Always remember to give self-care priority and schedule time for mental, physical, and spiritual well-being. Take part in things that make you happy, help you decompress, and improve your general well-being.

You can raise your chances of long-term success on the Blood Sugar Diet by establishing a solid support network and fostering an atmosphere that is in line with your health objectives. Recall that you don't have to travel this path alone and that it's acceptable to ask for assistance and support when you need it.

Chapter 8: Modifying Your Lifestyle for Long-Term Success

Advice on Changing Your Diet and Lifestyle in a Sustainable Way

Select complete, unprocessed foods: Emphasize including fruits, vegetables, lean meats, and whole grains in your meals. These meals offer vital nutrients and typically have less sugar.

Restrict your intake of processed meals and sugary beverages: These items frequently have added sugars, which can raise your blood sugar levels. Make an effort to consume less of them and choose healthier substitutes.

Consume balanced meals: Make sure your plate has the right amount of healthy fats, protein, and carbs. This can assist in maintaining steady energy levels throughout the day and help control blood sugar levels.

Portion control: Pay attention to the sizes of your meals to avoid overindulging. Stable blood sugar levels can also be maintained by eating smaller, more frequent meals.

Eat more foods high in fiber: Fiber slows down the bloodstream's absorption of sugar. To boost your intake of fiber, include foods like fruits, vegetables, whole grains, and legumes in your diet.

Preserve your hydration: Drink plenty of water all day long to keep hydrated. A healthy blood sugar level can be supported by adequate hydration.

Regular exercise: Exercise on a regular basis can help control blood sugar levels and enhance insulin sensitivity. Engage in things you enjoy and strive for at least 150 minutes of moderate-intensity exercise each week.

Control your stress: Prolonged tension can affect your blood sugar levels. Discover appropriate coping mechanisms for stress, such as hobbies, relaxation exercises, or asking loved ones for assistance.

Get adequate sleep: Since good sleep helps to control blood sugar levels, make it a priority. Aim for 7 to 9 hours of sleep per night by creating a regular sleep regimen.

Remember, for individualized counsel and direction catered to your particular requirements, it's crucial to speak with a medical professional or registered dietitian. They are able to offer you a diet plan that works for your lifestyle and health objectives.

Creating reasonable objectives and monitoring advancement

Of course! The secret to sticking to your blood sugar diet plan is to set reasonable targets and monitor your success. The following is what you can do:

Establish clear, measurable goals: Begin with tiny, manageable goals rather than aiming for a dramatic improvement. For instance, you could try eating more veggies or drinking fewer sugar-filled beverages.

Break it down: Break down your objectives into more manageable steps. This helps you maintain your motivation and makes them easier to handle. If your objective is to exercise on a daily basis, for example, begin by setting aside 10 minutes and work your way up to a longer session.

Use a notebook or app: Use a journal or a mobile app to record your meals, activity, and blood sugar readings. This enables you to track your development, spot trends, and make necessary corrections.

Honor significant anniversaries: Honor your victories along the road!

Reward yourself with something unrelated to food when you accomplish a goal, such as reading a new book or taking a relaxing spa day. This can apply to reaching weight loss milestones as well as stable blood sugar levels.

Find support: Get in the company of a positive support system. Tell your loved ones about your objectives, or join online groups to interact with people who are also controlling their blood sugar. Both accountability and support may make a big difference.

Frequent check-ins: Make an appointment with your registered dietician or healthcare provider on a frequent basis. They can offer advice, keep an eye on your development, and modify your food and lifestyle plan as needed.

Recall that it takes time to make progress, therefore you should practice self-compassion. Remain dedicated to bringing about long-lasting change while acknowledging the little wins.

Honoring Achievements and Overcoming Obstacles

A crucial component of your blood sugar diet solution journey is acknowledging and celebrating your accomplishments and conquering obstacles. You'll find the following guidance useful on your journey:

Celebrate your victories: Regardless of how minor they may appear, take a minute to recognize and honor your accomplishments. Give yourself a pat on the back and feel happy about your achievements, whether it's sticking to your diet plan for a week, completing a weight reduction milestone, or maintaining stable blood sugar levels.

Stay motivated: Remind yourself of the reasons you began this trip in order to maintain your motivation. Imagine how controlling your blood sugar levels can improve your general health and wellbeing. Embrace a community of like-minded individuals who will encourage and support you when you need it.

Be ready for obstacles: Remember that you're not alone when you encounter difficulties along the path. Plan ahead for probable roadblocks, such cravings or social circumstances, and devise countermeasures. One way to prepare ahead of time is to bring along nutritious snacks, look for alternatives when dining out, or consult a certified dietitian or other healthcare provider for assistance.

Learn from mistakes: Try not to punish yourself if you make mistakes or encounter difficulties. Consider them as opportunities for learning instead.

Consider what caused the setback and devise a plan of action to ensure it doesn't occur again. Recall that every day presents an opportunity for fresh start and that growth is not always linear.

Remain consistent: When it comes to controlling your blood sugar levels, consistency is essential. Adhere to your meal plan, get frequent exercise, and prioritize making good food choices. These routines will become second nature with time and help you succeed in the long run.

Remain informed: Keep abreast of the most recent findings and information about controlling blood sugar. This will assist you in making well-informed decisions on your lifestyle and eating. For individualized counsel and direction, speak with medical specialists or registered dietitians who focus on blood sugar control.

Recall that every step you take ahead is a step in the correct direction since you are changing for the better in terms of your health. Keep up the fantastic work.

Summary of the Blood Sugar Diet Solution's Important Points

The main ideas of the Blood Sugar Diet Resolution are summarized as follows:

Include whole foods: Make it a point to include unprocessed, entire foods in your diet. Fruits, vegetables, whole grains, lean meats, and healthy fats are a few of these. These foods support blood sugar regulation and offer vital nutrients.

Restrict processed foods and sugary drinks: Reduce the amount of processed foods you eat, including soda, refined grains, and sugary snacks. Blood sugar increases brought on by certain foods may result in weight gain.

Regular exercise: To assist control blood sugar levels and encourage weight loss, get moving regularly. Make an effort to include strength, flexibility,

Blood sugar diet solution

and cardiovascular conditioning in your regimen. Find out which workout program is best for you by speaking with a healthcare provider.

Portion control: Pay attention to the sizes of your meals to avoid overindulging. Use smaller bowls and plates and be aware of your body's signals of hunger and fullness. Blood sugar levels can be more easily controlled by eating smaller, more balanced meals throughout the day.

Preserve your hydration: Drink plenty of water all day long to keep hydrated. Restrict the amount of sugary drinks you consume because they may cause blood sugar to rise.

Seek assistance: Take into consideration attending a support group or consulting a medical expert or certified dietitian with expertise in blood sugar control. They can track your development, give you tailored guidance, and support you every step of the way.

Recall that the goals of the Blood Sugar Diet Solution are to support general health and assist in controlling blood sugar levels. Any major modifications to your diet or fitness regimen should be discussed with a healthcare provider beforehand. Personalized guidance can be provided based on your specific needs and medical history.

Motivation to Maintain Success in Blood Sugar Management

You're doing a fantastic job controlling your blood sugar! Maintain your excellent work by following the Blood Sugar Diet Solution. Recall to prioritize natural meals, minimize processed foods and sugar-filled beverages, and maintain an active lifestyle through consistent exercise. Your perseverance and effort will be rewarded, and I have faith in your ongoing success! Proceed! And never give up on yourself.